FOREWORD

The essence of nutrition guidance is to provide the public with the best information available to assist them in making wise and nutritious food choices to sustain life and good health. As public officials in the U.S. Department of Agriculture, we are deeply concerned that Americans not only have enough food but also that the public has enough information to know what food to purchase and how to prepare it.

While a healthy diet is the cornerstone to good health, meeting that goal can be a challenge. That is why we are delighted to offer this publication to the public. *Recipes and Tips for Healthy, Thrifty Meals* is more than a cookbook. The book provides basic cooking and food safety guidance. The menus presented here conform to the recommendations contained in the Dietary Guidelines for Americans and the USDA Food Guide Pyramid. The 40 recipes are quick, easy, tasty and economical.

We hope that you will find the recipes and other information provided in this book useful. At the back of the book is information on how to get more nutrition information. If you have comments or suggestions, let us hear from you.

Shirley R. Watkins
Shirley R. Watkins
Under Secretary
Food, Nutrition and
Consumer Services

Rajen S. Anand, Ph.D.
Executive Director
Center for Nutrition
Policy and Promotion

1

TABLE OF CONTENTS

INTRODUCTION

How can you serve healthy meals on a limited budget? It takes some time and planning, but you and your family can eat better for less. This booklet can help you save money as you prepare healthy meals. It contains

- Tips for planning, shopping, and cooking healthy meals on a tight budget
- Sample menus for 2 weeks for breakfast, lunch, dinner, and snacks
- Recipes for healthy, thrifty meals
- Lists of the foods needed for each weekly menu

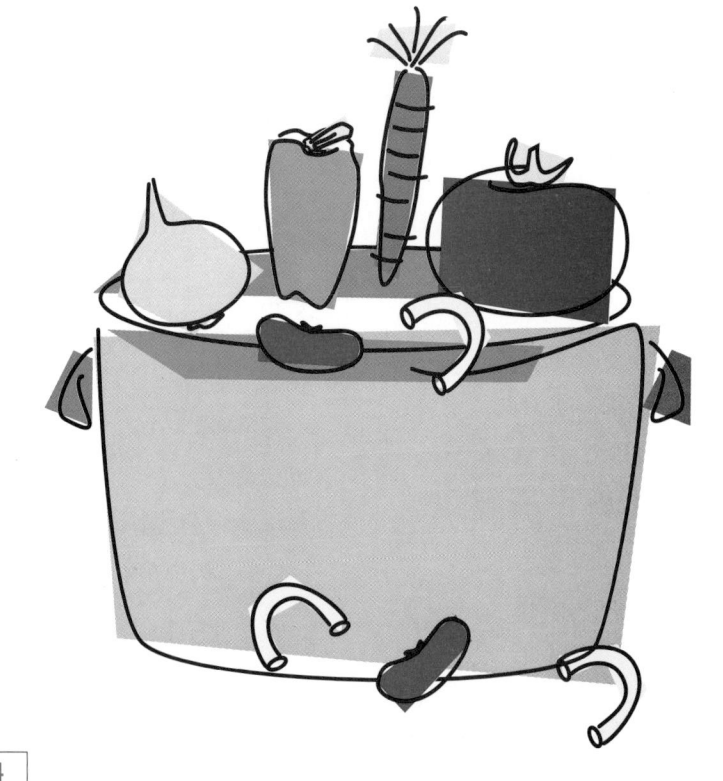

TIPS FOR HEALTHY, THRIFTY MEALS

WHY PLAN MEALS?

To help you and your family be healthier. When you plan meals, you can make sure you include enough foods from each food group. Pay special attention to serving enough vegetables and fruits in family meals.

To help you balance meals. When you are serving a food with a lot of fat or salt, you can plan lowfat or low-salt foods to go with it. For example, ham is high in salt. If you have ham for dinner, you also can serve a salad or a vegetable that doesn't need salt.

To save money. If you plan before you go food shopping, you will know what you have on hand and what you need. Also, shopping from a list helps you avoid expensive "impulse" purchases.

To save time and effort. When you plan meals, you have foods on hand and make fewer trips to the grocery store. Planning also helps you make good use of leftovers. This can cut your cooking time and food costs.

TIPS FOR PLANNING

Build the main part of your meal around rice, noodles, or other grains. Use small amounts of meat, poultry, fish, or eggs.

- For example, make a casserole by mixing rice, vegetables, and chicken. Or try Beef-Noodle Casserole (p. 22) or Stir-Fried Pork and Vegetables with Rice (p. 26).

Add variety to family meals. In addition to cooking family favorites, try new, low-cost recipes or food combinations.

- For example, if you usually serve mashed potatoes, try Baked Crispy Potatoes (p. 49) or Potato Salad (p. 58) for a change.

continued

Make meals easier to prepare by trying new ways to cook foods.

- For example, try using a slow cooker or crock-pot to cook stews or soups. They cook foods without constant watching.

Use planned leftovers to save both time and money.

- For example, prepare a Beef Pot Roast (p. 21), serve half of it, and freeze the remaining half to use later. You also can freeze extra cooked meats and vegetables for soups or stews.

Do "batch cooking" when your food budget and time allow.

- For example, cook a large batch of Baked Meatballs (p. 20) or Turkey Chili (p. 39), divide it into family-size portions, and freeze some for meals later in the month.

Plan snacks that give your family the nutrients they need.

- For example, buy fresh fruits in season like apples or peaches. Dried fruits like raisins or prunes, raw vegetables, crackers, and whole wheat bread are also good ideas for snacks.

TIPS FOR SHOPPING
Before you go shopping

- Make a list of all the foods you need. Do this in your kitchen so you can check what you have on hand.
- Look for specials in the newspaper ads for the stores where you shop.
- Look for coupons for foods you plan to buy. But remember, coupons save money only if you need the product. Also, check if other brands are on sale, too. They may cost even less than the one with a coupon.

continued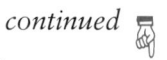

While you shop

- When your food budget allows, buy extra low-cost, nutritious foods like potatoes and frozen orange juice concentrate. These foods keep well.
- Compare the cost of convenience foods with the same foods made from scratch. "Convenience foods" are products like fancy baked goods, frozen meals, and vegetables with seasonings and sauces. Most of these cost more than similar foods prepared at home. Also, you can use less fat, sugar, and salt in food you make at home.
- Try store brands. They usually cost less than name brands, but they taste as good and generally have the same nutritional value.
- Take time to compare fresh, frozen, and canned foods to see which is cheapest. Buy what's on special and what's in season.
- Prevent food waste. Buy only the amount that your family will eat before the food spoils.

Using label and shelf information

- Read the Nutrition Facts label on packaged foods. Compare the amount of fat, sodium, calories, and other nutrients in similar products. This can help you choose foods that have less fat, sodium or calories, and more vitamins, minerals, and fiber.
- Use date information on packages—"sell by" and "best if used by" dates—to help you choose the freshest foods.
- Look for the unit price to compare similar foods. It tells you the cost per ounce, pound, or pint, so you'll know which brand or size is the best buy. Most stores show the unit price on a shelf sticker just below the product.

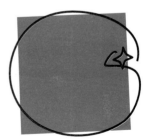

SOME BEST BUYS FOR COST AND NUTRITION

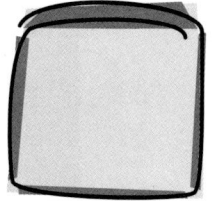

BREADS AND GRAINS

Look for bargains on day-old bread and bakery products.

Buy regular rice, oatmeal, and grits instead of the instant and flavored types.

Try whole-grain bread and brown rice to add nutrients and variety to family meals.

VEGETABLES AND SALADS

Look for large bags of frozen vegetables. They may be bargains and you can cook just the amount you need, close the bag tightly, and put the rest back in the freezer.

Foods at salad bars can be costly. Some food items—lettuce, cabbage, onions, and carrots—usually cost less in the produce section of the store than at the salad bar. But if you need only a small amount of a vegetable, buying at the salad bar can save money if it reduces the amount you waste.

FRUITS

Buy fresh fruits in season, when they generally cost less.

continued

MILK	Nonfat dry milk is the least expensive way to buy milk. When using it as a beverage, mix it several hours ahead and refrigerate so it can get cold before drinking.
	Buy fresh milk in large containers (gallon or 1/2 gallon). These generally cost less than quarts.
	Buy fat-free or lowfat milk to cut the amount of fat in your family's meals. Note that children under 2 years of age should be given only whole milk.
MEAT AND POULTRY	Look for specials at the meat counter. Buying cuts of meat on sale can mean big savings for you.
	Buy chuck or bottom round roast instead of sirloin. These cuts have less fat and cost less. They need to be covered during cooking and cooked longer to make the meat tender.
	Buy whole chickens and cut them into serving size pieces yourself.
DRY BEANS AND PEAS	Use these sometimes instead of meat, poultry, or fish. They cost less and provide many of the same nutrients. They are also lower in fat.
BULK FOODS	Buy bulk foods when they are available. They can be lower in price than similar foods sold in packages. Also, you can buy just the amount you need.

TIPS FOR HEALTHY COOKING

- Go easy on fat, sugar, and salt in preparing foods. For example, make Oven Crispy Chicken (p. 37) instead of fried chicken or make Baked Cod with Cheese (p. 28) instead of fried fish. You don't have to leave out all the fat, sugar, or salt—just limit the amount you use.
- Flavor foods with herbs, spices, and other lowfat seasonings instead of using rich sauces and gravy. Look for ideas about what seasonings to use in some of the recipes in this booklet, like Baked Meatballs (p. 20), Baked Spicy Fish (p. 29), and Turkey Chili (p. 39).
- Make homemade desserts sometimes to save money and serve additional healthy foods to the family. For example, try a fruit crisp, like Peach-Apple Crisp (p. 65), or a pudding like Rice Pudding (p. 67).
- Remove skin from poultry before cooking to lower the fat content. For example, try Baked Chicken Nuggets (p. 34), Chicken and Vegetables (p. 36), or Oven Crispy Chicken (p. 37).
- Always follow food safety rules in the kitchen to make sure that the food you prepare for your family is safe. See the next page.

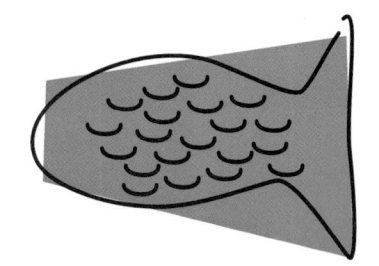

KEEP YOUR FAMILY'S FOOD SAFE

Clean—wash hands and surfaces often:
- Always wash hands with soap and warm running water before handling food.
- Always wash cutting boards, knives, utensils, dishes, and countertops used to cut meat with soapy, hot water right away—before you use them for other foods.
- Consider using paper towels to clean up kitchen surfaces. If you use cloth towels, dishcloths, or sponges, wash them often, and every time they have touched raw meat, poultry, or seafood juices. Use hot soapy water or the hot water cycle of the washing machine.

Separate—don't cross contaminate:
- Store raw meat, chicken, turkey, and seafood in a sealed, wrapped container in the refrigerator.
- Keep raw meat, chicken, turkey, and seafood away from foods that will not be cooked and foods that are already cooked.
- Never place cooked food on a plate or cutting board that previously held raw meat, chicken, turkey, or seafood.

Cook—cook to proper temperatures:
- Use a food thermometer to make sure meats, chicken, turkey, fish, and casseroles are cooked to a safe internal temperature.
  - Cook roasts and steaks to at least 145° F.
  - Cook ground meat to at least 160° F.
  - Cook whole chicken or turkey to 180° F.
- Cook eggs until the yolk and white are firm, not runny. Don't use recipes in which eggs remain raw or only partially cooked.
- Cook fish until it flakes easily with a fork.

continued

Chill—refrigerate promptly:

- Thaw frozen foods in the refrigerator, not on the kitchen counter. You can also thaw foods under cold water, changing the water every 30 minutes. Or, use a microwave oven.
- Refrigerate or freeze leftover foods right away. Meat, chicken, turkey, seafood, and egg dishes should not sit out at room temperature for more than 2 hours.
- Divide large amounts of leftovers into small, shallow containers for quick cooling in the refrigerator.
- Keep your refrigerator at 40°F or below. Don't pack the refrigerator. Cool air needs to circulate to keep food safe.

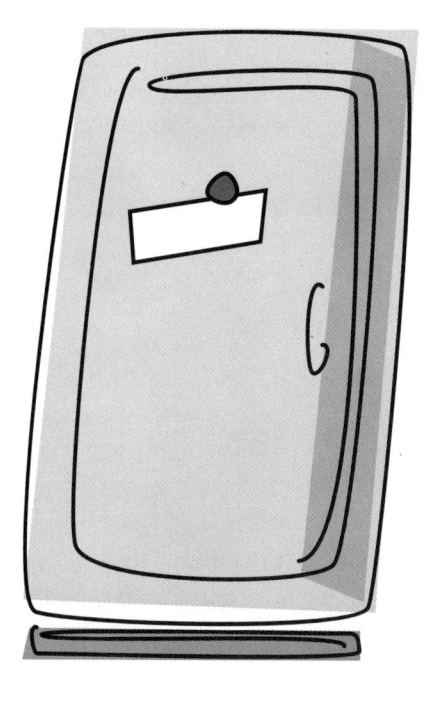

MENUS

These menus are not rigid guides and can be used in any order. They give suggestions for thrifty food choices and healthy ways to prepare foods. The foods used in the menus are a variety of commonly eaten meats, milk products, vegetables, fruits, grain products, and mixed dishes.

The daily menus show how you can combine a larger amount of less expensive foods, such as dry beans and grain products, with a smaller amount of meats, poultry, and fish. Some convenience or ready-to-eat food items are included in the menus. However, many of the foods are prepared from "scratch" to keep cost as low as possible.

These menus and recipes are designed for a healthy four-person family. The amount listed after each food item is the **total amount** for a family with two adults and two children 6 to 11 years old.

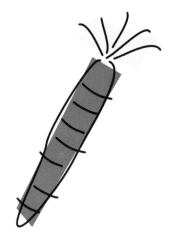

WEEK 1. MENUS FOR A FAMILY OF FOUR

	MONDAY	TUESDAY	WEDNESDAY	THURSDAY	FRIDAY	SATURDAY	SUNDAY

BREAKFAST	Orange juice (3 c)
	Ready-to-eat
	  cereal (3 c flakes)
	Toasted English
	  muffin (4)
	1% lowfat milk (2 c)
		Orange juice (3 c)
		Banana (4)
		Bagel (4)
		Margarine (4 tsp)
		1% lowfat milk (2 c)
			Orange juice (3 c)
			Cooked rice cereal
			Bagel (4)
			Margarine (4 tsp)
				Orange juice (3 c)
				Scrambled eggs (4)
				Hash brown
				  potatoes (2 c)
				1% lowfat milk (2 c)
					Orange juice (3 c)
					Ready-to-eat cereal
					  (3 c flakes)
					English muffin (4)
					Margarine (4 tsp)
					1% lowfat milk (2 c)
						Orange juice (3 c)
						Baked French toast
						Cinnamon sugar
						  topping (4 tsp)
						1% lowfat milk (2 c)
							Orange juice (3 c)
							Baked potato cakes
							White toast
							  (4 slices)
							1% lowfat milk (2 c)

LUNCH	Turkey patties
	Hamburger bun (4)
	Orange juice (3 c)
	Coleslaw (2 c)
	1% lowfat milk (2 c)
		Crispy chicken
		Potato salad
		Orange gelatin
		  salad
		Peaches, canned (1 c)
		Rice pudding
			Turkey chili
			Macaroni (2 c)
			Peach-apple crisp
			1% lowfat milk (2 c)
			Orange juice (3 c)
				Turkey ham (11 oz,
				  2 tbsp salad
				  dressing)
				  sandwiches (4)
				Baked beans
				Banana slices (2 c)
				Oatmeal cookies
				Orange juice (3 c)
				1% lowfat milk (2 c)
					Potato soup
					Snack crackers,
					  low salt (5 each)
					Tuna pasta salad
					Orange slices (2 c)
					Oatmeal cookies
					1% lowfat milk (2 c)
						Potato soup
						Snack crackers,
						  low salt (5 each)
						Apple orange slices
						  (2 apples,
						  2 oranges) (2 c)
						Rice pudding
						1% lowfat milk (2 c)
							Baked fish (12 oz,
							  4 tbsp salad
							  dressing)
							  sandwiches (4)
							Crispy potatoes
							Macaroni salad
							Melon (1-1/3 c)
							Orange juice (3 c)
							1% lowfat milk (2 c)

continued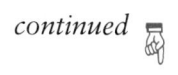

MONDAY	TUESDAY	WEDNESDAY	THURSDAY	FRIDAY	SATURDAY	SUNDAY
DINNER						
Beef-noodle casserole Lima beans (2 c) Banana orange salad (2 bananas, 2 oranges) (2 c) 1% lowfat milk (2 c)	Turkey stir fry Steamed rice (3 c) White bread (4 slices) Peach-apple crisp 1% lowfat milk (2 c)	Baked cod w/cheese Scalloped potatoes Spinach (1-1/3 c) Margarine (4 tsp) Chocolate pudding (2 c)	Beef pot roast Noodles (4 c) Peas and carrots (1 c) Orange slices (2 c) Biscuits (8) Margarine (4 tsp) Rice pudding 1% lowfat milk (2 c)	Beef pot roast (12 oz) Noodles (4 c) Green beans (1-1/3 c) Leaf lettuce (1-1/3 c) Salad dressing (4 tbsp) Rice pudding 1% lowfat milk (2 c)	Saucy beef pasta White bread (4) Canned pears (2 c) Orange juice (3 c) 1% lowfat milk (2 c)	Turkey-cabbage casserole (8 c) Orange slices (2 c) White bread (2 slices) Chickpea dip 1% lowfat milk (2 c)
SNACK						
White bread (4 slices) Chickpea dip Lemonade (4 c)	Orange juice (3 c)	Crispy potatoes	Lemonade (4 c)	Biscuits (8) Margarine (4 tsp) Lemonade (4 c)	Lemonade (4 c)	

Recipes are provided for foods in bold typeface.

WEEK II. MENUS FOR A FAMILY OF FOUR

	MONDAY	TUESDAY	WEDNESDAY	THURSDAY	FRIDAY	SATURDAY	SUNDAY

BREAKFAST	Orange juice (3 c)
	Hash brown
	  potatoes (2 c)
	Biscuits (8)
	Margarine (4 tsp)
	Jelly (8 tbsp)
		Orange juice (3 c)
		Ready-to-eat
		  cereal
		  (3 c toasted oats)
		White toast
		  (4 slices)
		Margarine (8tsp)
		1% lowfat milk (2c)
			Orange juice (3 c)
			Bananas (1/2 c)
			Ready-to-eat
			  cereal
			  (3 c toasted oats)
			White toast
			  (4 slices)
			Jelly (8 tbsp)
			1% lowfat milk (2 c)
				Orange juice (3 c)
				Cooked rice cereal
				White toast
				  (4 slices)
				Margarine (8 tsp)
				1% lowfat milk (2 c)
					Orange juice (3 c)
					Ready-to-eat
					  cereal
					  (3 c toasted oats)
					White toast
					  (4 slices)
					Margarine (4 tsp)
					1% lowfat milk (2 c)
						Orange juice (3 c)
						Scrambled eggs
						  (2 c)
						Turkey ham (11 oz)
						Bagels (4)
						1% lowfat milk (2 c)
							Orange juice (3 c)
							Melon (1-1/3 c)
							Pancakes (12)
							Pancake syrup
							  (8 tbsp)
							1% lowfat milk (2 c)

LUNCH	Chicken and
	  vegetables
	Scalloped potatoes
	Grapes (12 oz)
	Whole wheat bread
	  (4 slices)
	Margarine (4 tsp)
	Peach cake
	1% lowfat milk (2 c)
		Pizza meat loaf
		Noodles (4 c)
		Margarine (8 tsp)
		Orange slices (2 c)
		1% lowfat milk (2 c)
			Tuna macaroni
			  salad
			White bread
			  (4 slices)
			Margarine (4 tsp)
			Apple slices (2 c)
			1% lowfat milk (2 c)
			Cocoa drink mix
			  (2 oz)
				Hamburger (12 oz)
				  sandwiches (4)
				Ranch beans
				Orange gelatin
				  salad
				Banana slices (1/2 c)
				1% lowfat milk (2 c)
					Baked chicken
					  nuggets
					Shoestring potatoes
					Macaroni (5 c)
					Margarine (4 tsp)
					Orange gelatin
					  salad
					1% lowfat milk (2 c)
						Chicken noodle
						  soup
						Biscuits (8)
						Canned peaches
						  (2 c)
						Orange juice (3 c)
						1% lowfat milk (2 c)
						Cocoa drink mix
						  (2 oz)
							Meatball (12)
							  sandwiches (4)
							Grapes (12 oz)
							Sugar cookies
							1% lowfat milk (2 c)
							Orange juice (3 c)

continued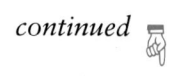

MONDAY	TUESDAY	WEDNESDAY	THURSDAY	FRIDAY	SATURDAY	SUNDAY
DINNER						
Southwestern salad	Spanish baked fish	Stir-fried pork and vegetables with rice	Baked chicken (10 oz)	Baked spicy fish	Baked meatballs	Cheese-stuffed potatoes
Steamed rice (6 c)	Steamed rice (6 c)	Dinner rolls (4)	Mash potatoes (6 c)	Noodles (4 c)	Spaghetti and sauce (5 c)	Macaroni (5 c)
Apple orange salad (2 apples, 2 oranges) (2 c)	Peas (1-1/3 c)	Margarine (4 tsp)	Green beans (1-1/2 c)	Peas and carrots (10 oz)	Leaf lettuce (2 c)	Peas (1-1/3 c)
Margarine (4 tsp)	Whole wheat bread (4 slices)	Mandarin oranges (2 c)	White bread (4 slices)	White bread (4 slices)	Salad dressing (4 tbsp)	Margarine (8 tsp)
1% lowfat milk (2 c)	Margarine (8 tsp)	1% lowfat milk (2 c)	Margarine (5-1/3 tbsp)	Margarine (8 tsp)	French bread (4 slices)	Orange slices (2 c)
	Peach cake		Orange slices (2 c)	Chocolate rice pudding	1% lowfat milk (2 c)	1% lowfat milk (2 c)
	1% lowfat milk (2 c)		1% lowfat milk (2 c)	1% lowfat milk (2 c)		
SNACK						
Popcorn (6 c)	Shoestring potatoes	Popcorn (6 c)	Chocolate rice pudding	Baked French fries (11 oz)	Ice milk fudgesicle (4)	Popcorn (6 c)
	Fruit drink (4 c)	Orange juice (3 c)		Fruit drink (4 c)		Fruit drink (4 c)

Recipes are provided for foods in bold typeface.

RECIPES

The following 40 recipes were developed for the 2 sample weekly menus. Many of them combine larger amounts of less expensive foods with smaller amounts of moderately priced foods. They also show how you can prepare tasty, healthy meals with less fat, sugar, and salt. Serve these recipes along with the other foods listed in each menu. You can also serve them in meals with other foods your family likes.

Each recipe lists
- ingredients and preparation instructions,
- the number of servings it will make,
- the size of each serving,
- the amount of preparation time,
- the amount of cooking time, and
- the calories, total fat, saturated fat, cholesterol, and sodium in a serving.

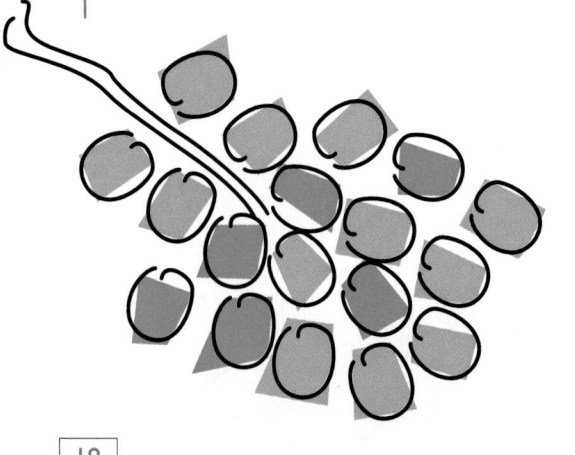

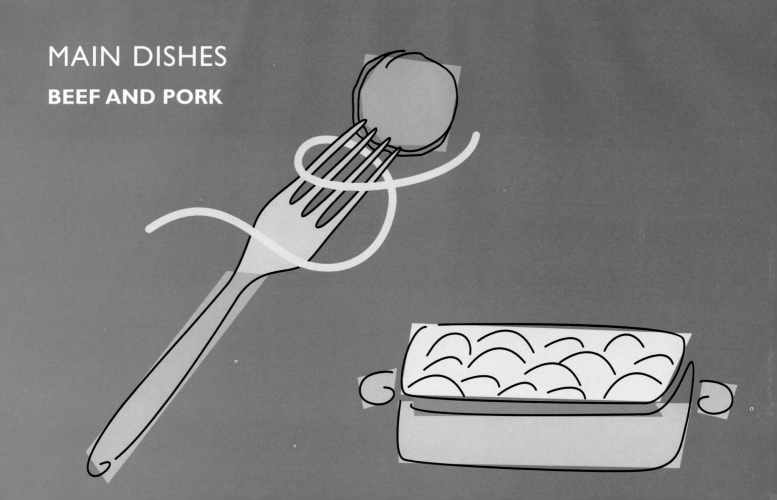

MAIN DISHES

BEEF AND PORK

BAKED MEATBALLS

4 Servings, about 3 meatballs each, plus 4 servings for another meal

Onions, minced	1/4 cup
Vegetable oil	1 tablespoon
Lean ground beef	2 pounds
Eggs	2
Bread crumb	3/4 cup
Whole milk	1/2 cup
Salt	1/8 teaspoon
Pepper	1/2 teaspoon
Onion powder	2 teaspoons
Garlic powder	1/2 teaspoon

PREPARATION TIME: 15 MINUTES
COOKING TIME: 10 TO 12 MINUTES

1. Preheat oven 400° F. Grease baking sheet lightly with oil.
2. Add 1 tablespoon oil and onions to small skillet. Cook over medium heat, until tender, about 3 minutes.
3. Mix remaining ingredients together in bowl; add onions. Mix until blended, using a large serving spoon.
4. Shape beef mixture into 1- to 2-inch meatballs; place on baking sheet.
5. Bake until thoroughly cooked, about 10 to 12 minutes.

Note: Serve with spaghetti sauce and in the meatball sandwich.

PER SERVING:	
Calories	345
Total fat	21 grams
Saturated fat	7 grams
Cholesterol	142 milligrams
Sodium	224 milligrams

BEEF POT ROAST

4 Servings, about 3 ounces beef each, plus 4 servings for another meal

Onion, chopped	1/2 cup
Water	2 tablespoons
Beef chuck roast, boneless	2-1/2 pounds
Hot water	2 cups
Beef bouillon	1 cube
Orange juice	2 tablespoons
Ground allspice	1/4 teaspoon
Pepper	1/8 teaspoon

PREPARATION TIME: 20 MINUTES
COOKING TIME: 2 HOURS

1. Simmer onion until tender in 2 tablespoons water in heavy, deep skillet.
2. Add roast to skillet; brown on sides.
3. Combine beef bouillon cube with 2 cups hot water; stir until dissolved.
4. Combine orange juice, allspice, pepper, and beef broth. Pour over meat. Cover and simmer, about 2 hours.

PER SERVING:

Calories	220
Total fat	9 grams
Saturated fat	3 grams
Cholesterol	91 milligrams
Sodium	264 milligrams

BEEF-NOODLE CASSEROLE

4 Servings, about 2 cups each

Lean ground beef	1 pound
Onions, chopped finely	1/2 cup
Boiling water	3 quarts
Noodles, yolk-free, enriched, uncooked	2-3/4 cups
Tomato soup, condensed	1 10-3/4-ounce can
Water	1-1/4 cups
Pepper	1/8 teaspoon
Bread crumbs	1 cup

PREPARATION TIME: 20 MINUTES
COOKING TIME: 30 MINUTES

1. Brown beef and onions in hot skillet; drain.
2. Place water in large saucepan; bring to rolling boil. Cook noodles in boiling water for 10 minutes; drain and set aside.
3. Combine soup, water, and pepper. Stir into cooked meat. Add cooked noodles to meat mixture. Stir gently to avoid tearing the noodles.
4. Spoon beef-noodle mixture into 9- by 13-inch baking pan. Sprinkle bread crumbs over beef-noodle mixture.
5. Bake, uncovered, at 300° F, about 30 minutes.

PER SERVING:

Calories	595
Total fat	18 grams
Saturated fat	6 grams
Cholesterol	86 milligrams
Sodium	575 milligrams

PIZZA MEAT LOAF

4 Servings, about 1/4 loaf each

Ground turkey	1 pound
Spaghetti sauce	3/4 cup
Mozzarella cheese, part-skim	1/4 cup
Green peppers, chopped	1/2 cup
Onion, minced	1/4 cup

PREPARATION TIME: 15 MINUTES
CONVENTIONAL COOKING TIME: 20 MINUTES
MICROWAVE COOKING TIME: 8 MINUTES

1. Lightly grease 9-inch pie plate with vegetable oil. Pat turkey into pie plate.

CONVENTIONAL METHOD

1. Place turkey in 350° F oven; bake until turkey no longer remains pink, about 17 to 20 minutes.

MICROWAVE METHOD

1. Cover turkey with waxed paper.
2. Cook on high; rotate plate 1/4 turn after 3 minutes.
3. Cook until turkey no longer remains pink, about 5 more minutes. Drain.

TO COMPLETE COOKING

1. Top baked turkey with spaghetti sauce, cheese, and vegetables.
2. Return turkey to either the conventional oven or the microwave oven and heat until cheese is melted, about 1 to 2 minutes.

PER SERVING:	
Calories	255
Total fat	14 grams
Saturated fat	4 grams
Cholesterol	88 milligrams
Sodium	376 milligrams

SAUCY BEEF PASTA

4 Servings, about 1-1/2 cups each

Water	1/2 cup
Green beans, frozen	1/2 10-ounce package
Onions, minced	1/2 cup
Lean ground beef	1 pound + 6 ounces
Noodles, yolk-free, enriched, uncooked	6-3/4 cups
Cold water	2 cups
Beef bouillon	2 cubes
Flour	1/3 cup
Pepper	1/4 teaspoon
Dry parsley flakes	1 teaspoon
Garlic powder	1/2 teaspoon
Onion powder	1 teaspoon

PREPARATION TIME: 25 MINUTES
COOKING TIME: ABOUT 35 MINUTES

1. Place 1/2 cup of water in saucepan. Cover and bring to boil. Add green beans, lower heat, and simmer until tender, about 5 minutes. Drain.

2. Place onions and ground beef in skillet. Cook over medium heat; stir occasionally. Cook until beef no longer remains pink, about 5 to 10 minutes. Drain fat off.

3. Cook noodles according to package instructions. Drain.

4. Combine cold water and flour; stir until smooth. Add flour mixture and beef bouillon cubes to ground beef. Cook, stirring frequently until mixture has thickened and bouillon cubes have dissolved, about 4 minutes.

5. Add cooked green beans, cooked noodles, pepper, parsley flakes, garlic powder, and onion powder to ground beef mixture; stir to combine.

6. Place beef mixture in 8- by 12-inch baking pan; cover and bake in 350° F oven until thoroughly heated, about 15 minutes.

PER SERVING:

Calories	605
Total fat	22 grams
Saturated fat	8 grams
Cholesterol	120 milligrams
Sodium	405 milligrams

SOUTHWESTERN SALAD

4 Servings, about 1/2 cup beef mixture, 1/2 cup lettuce and cheese mixture each

Onions, chopped	1/2 cup
Lean ground beef	1 pound
Chili powder	1 tablespoon
Dry oregano	2 teaspoons
Ground cumin	1/2 teaspoon
Canned kidney beans, red, drained	1 cup
Canned chickpeas, drained	1 15-ounce can
Tomato, diced	1 medium
Lettuce	2 cups
Cheddar cheese	1/2 cup

PREPARATION TIME: 15 MINUTES
COOKING TIME: 10 TO 15 MINUTES

1. Cook ground beef and onions in a large skillet until the beef no longer remains pink. Drain.
2. Stir chili powder, oregano, and cumin into beef mixture; cook for 1 minute.
3. Add beans, chickpeas, and tomatoes. Mix gently to combine.
4. Combine lettuce and cheese in large serving bowl. Portion lettuce and cheese onto 4 plates. Add 1 cup of beef mixture on top of lettuce and cheese.

Note: Garbanzo bean is another name for chickpea.

PER SERVING:

Calories	485
Total fat	22 grams
Saturated fat	9 grams
Cholesterol	98 milligrams
Sodium	411 milligrams

STIR-FRIED PORK AND VEGETABLES WITH RICE

4 Servings of pork and vegetables, about 1/2 cup each. 4 Servings of cooked rice, about 2 cups each

Chicken broth, reduced sodium	2 cups
Hot water	2 cups
Rice, uncooked	2 cups
Vegetable oil	2 tablespoons
Broccoli cuts, frozen	2 cups
Carrots, cleaned, sliced thinly	1 cup
Onions, minced	1/4 cup
Garlic powder	1 teaspoon
Canned mushrooms, drained	1/2 cup
Ground pork	1 pound + 7 ounces
Soy sauce	4 tablespoons

PREPARATION TIME: 20 MINUTES
COOKING TIME: 25 TO 30 MINUTES

1. Heat broth and water to a boil in sauce pan; add rice and return to boil. Reduce heat to low and simmer until tender, about 15 minutes.

2. Heat 1 tablespoon of oil in skillet. Add broccoli, carrots, onions, and garlic powder. Cook until crisp-tender, about 5 minutes. Remove from skillet. Add mushrooms. Cook for 1 minute and set aside.

3. Heat second tablespoon of oil in skillet. Add pork; cook until pork no longer remains pink. Drain liquid.

4. Add soy sauce and stir until mixed; add vegetables to pork mixture. Cook until heated, about 1 to 2 minutes.

5. Serve pork mixture over cooked rice.

Note: Sodium level can be reduced from 799 milligrams to 532 milligrams by reducing soy sauce from 4 to 2 tablespoons.

PER SERVING:	
Calories	860
Total fat	33 grams
Saturated fat	10 grams
Cholesterol	108 milligrams
Sodium	799 milligrams

MAIN DISHES

FISH

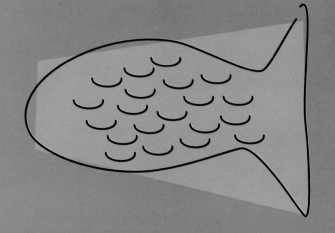

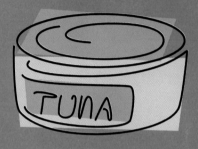

BAKED COD WITH CHEESE

4 Servings, about 3 ounces each

Cod fillets, fresh or frozen	1 pound
Cheddar cheese, shredded	4 tablespoons

PREPARATION TIME: 7 MINUTES
COOKING TIME: 15 MINUTES

1. Thaw cod according to package directions.

2. Prepare cod according to package directions.

3. After cod is fully cooked, sprinkle cheese on cod. Return cod to oven to melt cheese, about 3 to 5 minutes.

PER SERVING:

Calories	155
Total fat	5 grams
Saturated fat	3 grams
Cholesterol	65 milligrams
Sodium	160 milligrams

BAKED SPICY FISH

4 Servings, about 3 ounces each

Cod fillets, fresh or frozen	1 pound
Paprika	1/4 teaspoon
Garlic powder	1/4 teaspoon
Onion powder	1/4 teaspoon
Pepper	1/8 teaspoon
Ground oregano	1/8 teaspoon
Ground thyme	1/8 teaspoon
Lemon juice	1 tablespoon
Margarine, melted	1-1/2 tablespoons

PREPARATION TIME: 15 MINUTES
COOKING TIME: 25 MINUTES

1. Thaw frozen fish according to package directions.
2. Preheat oven to 350° F.
3. Separate fish into four fillets or pieces. Place fish in ungreased 13- by 9- by 2-inch baking pan.
4. Combine paprika, garlic and onion powder, pepper, oregano, and thyme in small bowl. Sprinkle seasoning mixture and lemon juice evenly over fish. Drizzle margarine evenly over fish.
5. Bake until fish flakes easily with a fork, about 20 to 25 minutes.

PER SERVING:	
Calories	140
Total fat	5 grams
Saturated fat	1 gram
Cholesterol	51 milligrams
Sodium	123 milligrams

29

SPANISH BAKED FISH

4 Servings, about 3 ounces each

Perch fillets, fresh or frozen	1 pound
Tomato sauce	1 cup
Onions, sliced	1/2 cup
Garlic powder	1/2 teaspoon
Chili powder	2 teaspoons
Dried oregano flakes	1 teaspoon
Ground cumin	1/8 teaspoon

PREPARATION TIME: 15 MINUTES
COOKING TIME: ABOUT 10 TO 20 MINUTES

1. Thaw frozen fish according to package directions.
2. Preheat oven to 350° F. Lightly grease baking dish.
3. Separate fish into four fillets or pieces. Arrange fish in baking dish.
4. Mix remaining ingredients together and pour over fish.
5. Bake until fish flakes easily with fork, about 10 to 20 minutes.

PER SERVING:

Calories	135
Total fat	1 gram
Saturated fat	Trace
Cholesterol	104 milligrams
Sodium	448 milligrams

TUNA MACARONI SALAD

4 Servings, about 1-1/2 cups each

Elbow macaroni, uncooked	1 cup
Canned tuna, water-pack, drained	2 6-ounce cans
Eggs, hard cooked, finely diced	4
Celery, chopped	1/4 cup
Carrots, grated	3/4 cup
Salad dressing, mayonnaise-type	1/2 cup
Onion, minced	2 tablespoons
Pepper	1/4 teaspoon

PREPARATION TIME: 15 MINUTES
COOKING TIME: 8 TO 10 MINUTES

1. Place water in large saucepan and bring to boil. Add macaroni and cook until tender, about 6 to 8 minutes. Drain.

2. Combine macaroni, tuna, eggs, celery, and carrots in a large bowl.

3. Stir together salad dressing, onion, and pepper. Spoon dressing over salad; toss until evenly combined.

4. Chill until ready to serve.

PER SERVING:

Calories	520
Total fat	30 grams
Saturated fat	5 grams
Cholesterol	237 milligrams
Sodium	509 milligrams

TUNA PASTA SALAD

4 Servings, about 1-1/2 cups each

Macaroni, uncooked	2 cups
Tuna, canned, water-pack	2 6-1/2-ounce cans
Zucchini, chopped	1/2 cup
Carrots, sliced	1/4 cup
Onions, diced	1/3 cup
Salad dressing, mayonnaise-type	1/4 cup

PREPARATION TIME: 25 MINUTES
COOKING TIME: 8 MINUTES

1. Cook macaroni according to package directions. Drain.

2. Drain tuna.

3. Wash vegetables. Chop zucchini; slice carrots into thin slices; dice onions.

4. Mix macaroni, tuna, and vegetables together in mixing bowl. Stir in salad dressing.

5. Chill until ready to serve.

PER SERVING:

Calories	405
Total fat	13 grams
Saturated fat	2 grams
Cholesterol	25 milligrams
Sodium	360 milligrams

MAIN DISHES

POULTRY

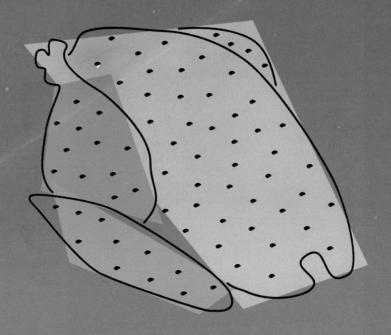

BAKED CHICKEN NUGGETS

4 Servings, about 3 ounces each

Chicken thighs, boneless, skinless	1-1/2 pounds
Ready-to-eat cereal, cornflakes, crumbs	1 cup
Paprika	1 teaspoon
Italian herb seasoning	1/2 teaspoon
Garlic powder	1/4 teaspoon
Onion powder	1/4 teaspoon

PREPARATION TIME: 15 MINUTES
CONVENTIONAL COOKING TIME: 12 TO 14 MINUTES
MICROWAVE COOKING TIME: 6 TO 8 MINUTES

1. Remove skin and bone; cut thighs into bite-sized pieces.
2. Place cornflakes in plastic bag and crush by using a rolling pin.
3. Add remaining ingredients to crushed cornflakes. Close bag tightly and shake until blended.
4. Add a few chicken pieces at a time to crumb mixture. Shake to coat evenly.

CONVENTIONAL METHOD

1. Preheat oven to 400° F. Lightly grease a cooking sheet.
2. Place chicken pieces on cooking sheet so they are not touching.
3. Bake until golden brown, about 12 to 14 minutes.

continued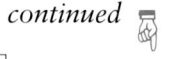

MICROWAVE METHOD:

1. Lightly grease an 8- by 12-inch baking dish.
2. Place chicken pieces on baking dish so they are not touching. Cover with waxed paper and cook on high.
3. Rotate chicken every 2 to 3 minutes. Cook until tender, about 6 to 8 minutes.

Note: To remove bone from chicken thighs:

1. Place chicken on cutting board. Remove skin from thighs.
2. Turn chicken thighs over.
3. Cut around bone and remove it.

PER SERVING:

Calories	175
Total fat	8 grams
Saturated fat	2 grams
Cholesterol	67 milligrams
Sodium	127 milligrams

CHICKEN AND VEGETABLES

4 Servings, about 1 cup each

Margarine	1-1/2 tablespoons
Garlic powder	1 teaspoon
Onions, chopped	1/2 cup
Chicken thighs, boneless, skinless	1 pound + 4 ounces
Cut green beans, frozen	10-ounce package
Pepper	1/4 teaspoon

PREPARATION TIME: 6 MINUTES
COOKING TIME: 25 MINUTES

1. Melt margarine in heavy skillet. Add garlic and onions; stir until blended. Cook over medium heat, until tender, about 5 minutes. Remove from skillet.

2. Place chicken in the skillet. Cook over medium heat, until chicken is thoroughly done and no longer pink in color, about 12 minutes. Remove chicken from skillet; keep warm.

3. Place frozen green beans, pepper, and cooked onions in same skillet. Cover and cook over medium-low heat until beans are tender, about 5 minutes.

4. Add chicken to vegetable mixture. Continue cooking, stirring occasionally, until heated through, about 3 minutes.

Note: To remove bone from chicken thighs:

1. Place chicken on cutting board. Remove skin from thighs.

2. Turn chicken thighs over.

3. Cut around bone and remove it.

PER SERVING:	
Calories	190
Total fat	11 grams
Saturated fat	3 grams
Cholesterol	57 grams
Sodium	109 milligrams

OVEN CRISPY CHICKEN

4 Servings, about 4 ounces each

Broiler fryer chicken, cut-up	1 1/2 pounds
Whole milk	1/4 cup
Flour	1/2 cup
Paprika	1 teaspoon
Pepper	1/2 teaspoon
Ready-to-eat flake cereal, slightly crushed	1 cup
Vegetable oil	4 tablespoons

PREPARATION TIME: 15 MINUTES
COOKING TIME: 30 MINUTES

1. Remove skin and all visible fat from chicken. Place milk in large bowl. Add chicken pieces; turn to coat.

2. Combine flour, paprika, and pepper on a plate.

3. Lift chicken pieces from milk and reserve milk. Coat chicken thoroughly with seasoned flour and place on a wire rack until all pieces have been coated. Redip chicken pieces into reserved milk.

4. Place crushed cereal on plate. Place chicken pieces on crushed cereal. Using 2 forks, turn chicken pieces in crushed cereal to coat.

5. Place chicken on a foil-lined baking tray; drizzle oil over chicken.

6. Bake at 400° F, for 15 minutes. Turn chicken pieces over; continue to bake until chicken is thoroughly cooked and crust is crisp, about 15 more minutes.

PER SERVING:	
Calories	350
Total fat	15 grams
Saturated fat	4 grams
Cholesterol	93 milligrams
Sodium	503 milligrams

TURKEY-CABBAGE CASSEROLE

4 Servings, about 2 cups each

Cabbage, shredded	1 cup
Ground turkey	1 pound
Onions, chopped	1/2 cup
White rice, uncooked	1 cup
Tomato sauce	2 cups
Garlic powder	1/2 teaspoon
Ground oregano	1/2 teaspoon

PREPARATION TIME: 10 MINUTES
COOKING TIME: 60 MINUTES

1. Place shredded cabbage in a lightly greased 2-quart casserole dish.
2. In skillet cook turkey until browned and no longer pink in color. Add chopped onions; stir occasionally and cook 3 minutes. Add uncooked rice to cooked turkey.
3. Place turkey-rice mixture over cabbage in casserole dish.
4. Combine tomato sauce, garlic, and oregano. Pour over cooked turkey.
5. Cover and bake at 350° F, about 1 hour.

PER SERVING:	
Calories	380
Total fat	11 grams
Saturated fat	3 grams
Cholesterol	77 milligrams
Sodium	829 milligrams

TURKEY CHILI

4 Servings, about 1-1/2 cups each

Ground turkey	1 pound
Onion, minced	3/4 cup
Margarine	2 tablespoons
Water	3 cups
Garlic powder	1/2 teaspoon
Chili powder	1 tablespoon
Dry parsley flakes	1 tablespoon
Paprika	1 teaspoon
Dry mustard	2 teaspoons
Canned red kidney beans, drained	1 15-1/2-ounce can
Tomato paste	1 6-ounce can
Pearl barley	1/2 cup
Cheddar cheese, shredded	3/4 cup

PREPARATION TIME: 30 MINUTES
COOKING TIME: 70 MINUTES

1. In large sauce pan, cook turkey and onions in margarine until turkey is browned and no longer pink in color, about 9 minutes. Drain; return turkey and onions to pan.

2. Add remaining ingredients except the cheese to turkey mixture; bring to boil, stirring frequently. Cover, reduce heat, and simmer 30 minutes, stirring occasionally.

3. Uncover and simmer 30 minutes, stirring occasionally.

4. Serve over cooked macaroni.

5. Sprinkle 3 tablespoons of cheese over each serving of chili.

PER SERVING:

Calories	540
Total fat	26 grams
Saturated fat	9 grams
Cholesterol	104 milligrams
Sodium	579 milligrams

TURKEY STIRFRY

4 Servings, about 1/2 cup each

Chicken bouillon cube	1
Hot water	1/2 cup
Soy sauce	2 tablespoons
Cornstarch	1 tablespoon
Vegetable oil	2 tablespoons
Garlic powder	1/2 teaspoon
Turkey, cubed	1 pound
Carrots, thinly sliced	1-3/4 cups
Zucchini, sliced	1 cup
Onions, thinly sliced	1/2 cup
Hot water	1/4 cup

PREPARATION TIME: 15 MINUTES
COOKING TIME: 10 MINUTES

1. Combine chicken bouillon cube and hot water to make broth; stir until dissolved.

2. Combine broth, soy sauce, and cornstarch in small bowl. Set aside.

3. Heat oil in skillet over high heat. Add garlic and turkey. Cook, stirring, until turkey is thoroughly cooked and no longer pink in color.

4. Add carrots, zucchini, onion, and water to cooked turkey. Cover and cook, stirring occasionally, until vegetables are tender-crisp, about 5 minutes. Uncover, bring turkey mixture to boil. Cook until almost all liquid has evaporated.

5. Stir in cornstarch mixture. Bring to boil, stirring constantly until thickened.

Note: Serve over steamed rice.

PER SERVING:	
Calories	195
Total fat	9 grams
Saturated fat	2 grams
Cholesterol	44 milligrams
Sodium	506 milligrams

TURKEY PATTIES

4 Servings, 1 patty each

Ground turkey	1 pound + 4 ounces
Bread crumbs	1 cup
Egg	1
Green onions, chopped	1/4 cup
Prepared mustard	1 tablespoon
Margarine	1-1/2 tablespoons
Chicken broth	1/2 cup

PREPARATION TIME: 15 MINUTES
COOKING TIME: 10 MINUTES

1. Mix ground turkey, bread crumbs, egg, onions, and mustard in large bowl. Shape into 4 patties, about 1/2-inch thick.

2. Melt margarine in large skillet over low heat. Add patties and cook, turning once to brown other side. Cook until golden brown outside and white inside, about 10 minutes. Remove from skillet and place onto plate.

3. Add chicken broth to skillet, and boil over high heat until slightly thickened, about 1 to 2 minutes. Pour sauce over patties.

4. Serve on buns.

PER SERVING:

Calories	305
Total fat	18 grams
Saturated fat	5 grams
Cholesterol	149 milligrams
Sodium	636 milligrams

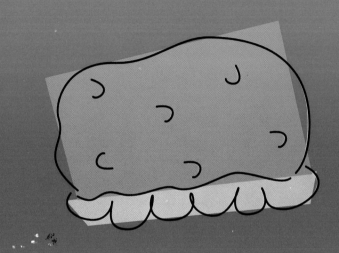

MAIN DISHES
VEGETARIAN

CHEESE-STUFFED POTATOES

4 Servings, two potato halves each

Baking potatoes	4 (8 ounces each)
Lowfat cottage cheese	7/8 cup
Whole milk	2 tablespoons
Onion, minced	2 tablespoons
Paprika	1/4 teaspoon

PREPARATION TIME: 20 MINUTES
CONVENTIONAL COOKING TIME: 30 TO 45 MINUTES
MICROWAVE COOKING TIME: 5 TO 10 MINUTES

1. Scrub potatoes and remove any blemishes.

TO BAKE:
CONVENTIONAL METHOD:

1. Preheat oven to 400° F.
2. Place potatoes in oven and bake until tender, about 30 to 40 minutes.

MICROWAVE METHOD:

1. Pierce potatoes by using fork prongs.
2. Cover potatoes with waxed paper. Heat on high until tender, about 5 to 10 minutes.

TO STUFF POTATOES:

1. Slice each potato in half, lengthwise. Using a spoon, scoop out pulp, leaving about 1/4-inch thick shells, saving pulp.
2. Blend cheese, milk, and onion. Add potato pulp; mix until light and fluffy.
3. Fill potato halves with mixture. Sprinkle paprika over potatoes.

Note: Return to oven or microwave to reheat, for a few minutes, if desired.

PER SERVING:	
Calories	250
Total fat	1 gram
Saturated fat	1 gram
Cholesterol	5 milligrams
Sodium	216 milligrams

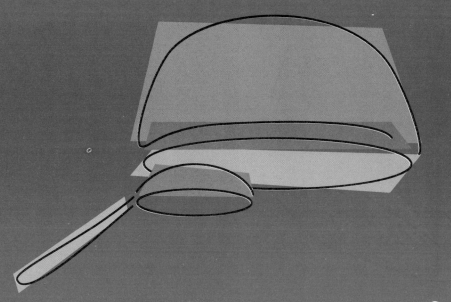

SOUPS

CHICKEN NOODLE SOUP

4 Servings, about 1-1/2 cups each, plus 4 servings for another meal

Vegetable oil	1 teaspoon
Onion, minced	1/2 cup
Carrots, diced	1/2 cup
Celery, sliced	1/2 cup
Garlic powder	1/2 teaspoon
Flour	1/8 cup
Dried oregano flakes	1/4 teaspoon
Chicken broth, reduced sodium	3 cups
Potatoes, peeled, diced	2 cups
Chicken, cooked, chopped	1/4 cup
Whole milk	1/2 cup
Noodles, yolk-free, enriched, uncooked	1 cup

PREPARATION TIME: 25 MINUTES
COOKING TIME: 35 TO 40 MINUTES

1. Heat oil over medium heat in large sauce pan. Add minced onions, carrots, celery, and garlic powder. Cook until onions are tender, about 3 to 5 minutes.

2. Sprinkle flour and oregano over vegetables; cook about 1 minute.

3. Stir in chicken broth and potatoes. Cover and cook until tender, about 20 minutes.

4. Add chicken, milk, and noodles. Cover and simmer until noodles are tender, about 10 minutes.

PER SERVING:	
Calories	205
Total fat	4 grams
Saturated fat	1 grams
Cholesterol	8 milligrams
Sodium	107 milligrams

POTATO SOUP

4 Servings, about 1 cup each, plus 4 servings for another meal

Onion, chopped	3/4 cup (1 medium)
Potatoes, peeled, diced	4-1/2 cups
Margarine	1 tablespoon
Flour	3 tablespoons
Whole milk	1 quart

PREPARATION TIME: 25 MINUTES
COOKING TIME: 15 MINUTES

1. Place onions and potatoes in sauce pan. Cover with water and bring to boil. Simmer until soft, about 10 minutes. Drain.

2. Melt margarine in saucepan. Add flour and stir until smooth. Heat to thicken.

3. Add onions and potatoes to milk mixture, and heat to serving temperature.

PER SERVING:

Calories	190
Total fat	6 grams
Saturated fat	3 grams
Cholesterol	17 milligrams
Sodium	325 milligrams

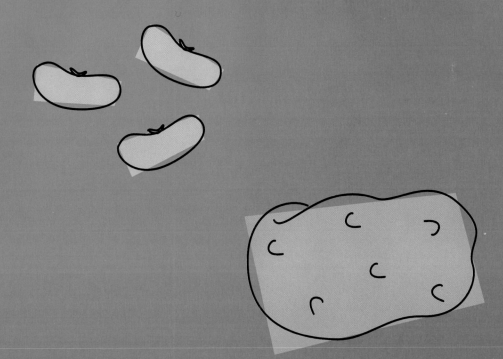

BAKED BEANS

4 Servings, about 3/4 cup each

Canned vegetarian beans	3 cups
Catsup	1/4 cup
Brown sugar	2 tablespoons

PREPARATION TIME: 5 MINUTES
COOKING TIME: 30 MINUTES

1. In small (1 quart) casserole dish, combine beans, catsup, and brown sugar.
2. Cover and bake at 350° F until bubbly, about minutes.

PER SERVING:	
Calories	220
Total fat	1 gram
Saturated fat	Trace
Cholesterol	0
Sodium	937 milligrams

BAKED CRISPY POTATOES

4 Servings, about 1/2 cup each, plus 4 servings for snack

Potatoes	4 pounds
Vegetable oil	4 tablespoons
Ground cumin	1 teaspoon
Red pepper	1/4 teaspoon

PREPARATION TIME: 10 MINUTES
COOKING TIME: 20 MINUTES

1. Lightly coat a 7- by 12- by 1-inch pan with oil.
2. Wash potatoes; cut in half lengthwise.
3. Place cut sides of potatoes on the oiled pan; rub potatoes in the oil; turn potatoes over so that cut sides are facing up.
4. Mix cumin and red pepper together; sprinkle over potatoes.
5. Bake at 400° F until potatoes are golden brown and tender, about 20 minutes.

PER SERVING:	
Calories	170
Total fat	5 grams
Saturated fat	1 gram
Cholesterol	0
Sodium	10 milligrams

POTATO CAKES

4 Servings, 1 cake each

New potatoes, cooked, peeled, mashed	2 cups
Egg	1
Flour	1 tablespoon
Whole milk	2 tablespoons
Vegetable oil	1/4 cup

PREPARATION TIME: 10 MINUTES
COOKING TIME: 5 MINUTES

1. Mix mashed potatoes, egg, flour, and milk thoroughly.
2. Shape into flat cakes, about 1/2-inch thick.
3. Heat oil in skillet.
4. Add potato cakes to hot skillet. Cook until golden brown and thoroughly heated.

PER SERVING:

Calories	210
Total fat	15 grams
Saturated fat	3 grams
Cholesterol	54 milligrams
Sodium	222 milligrams

RANCH BEANS

4 Servings, about 1 cup each

Green pepper, chopped	1/4 cup
Canned vegetarian beans	1-3/4 cups
Canned kidney beans, red, drained	1-3/4 cups
Catsup	2 tablespoons
Molasses	2 tablespoons
Dried onion	1/2 teaspoon

PREPARATION TIME: 5 MINUTES
COOKING TIME: 5 TO 10 MINUTES

CONVENTIONAL METHOD:

1. Place all ingredients in saucepan and heat thoroughly, about 10 minutes.

MICROWAVE METHOD:

1. Place all ingredients in microwave-safe bowl. Cover with waxed paper. Cook on high; stirring every 2 minutes; cook about 5 minutes.

PER SERVING:

Calories	240
Total fat	1 gram
Saturated fat	Trace
Cholesterol	0
Sodium	916 milligrams

SCALLOPED POTATOES

4 Servings, about 1-1/2 cups each

Potatoes	2 pounds
Margarine	2 tablespoons
Onions, sliced	1 cup
Flour	3 tablespoons
Pepper	1/4 teaspoon
Whole milk	2 cups

PREPARATION TIME: 20 MINUTES
COOKING TIME: 15 MINUTES

1. Wash potatoes; peel and slice into thin slices.
2. Melt 1 tablespoon of margarine in heavy, deep skillet. Remove skillet from heat; spread half of potato slices in skillet.
3. Cover potatoes with onions. Sprinkle half of flour and pepper over potato mixture.
4. Add remaining potato slices, flour, and pepper. Cut 1 tablespoon of margarine into small pieces and place on top of potato mixture.
5. Pour milk over potato mixture; bring to boil over high heat. Reduce heat to medium low, cover, and cook until potatoes are tender, about 15 minutes.

PER SERVING:

Calories	305
Total fat	10 grams
Saturated fat	4 grams
Cholesterol	17 milligrams
Sodium	139 milligrams

SHOESTRING POTATOES

4 Servings, about 6 ounces each

Potatoes	1-1/2 pounds
Vegetable oil	3 tablespoons
Salt	1/4 teaspoon
Pepper	1/4 teaspoon

PREPARATION TIME: 15 MINUTES
COOKING TIME: 30 MINUTES

1. Preheat oven to 450° F.
2. Wash potatoes; cut lengthwise into thin strips.
3. Combine remaining ingredients in plastic bag. Put potatoes in bag; seal; shake to coat potatoes.
4. Arrange potatoes in single layer on baking sheet.
5. Bake until crisp and golden, about 30 minutes.

PER SERVING:

Calories	255
Total fat	14 grams
Saturated fat	2 grams
Cholesterol	0
Sodium	156 milligrams

CHICKPEA DIP

4 Servings, about 3 tablespoons each, plus 4 servings for another meal or snack.

Canned chickpeas, drained	1 15-1/2-ounce can
Vegetable oil	2 tablespoons
Lemon juice	1 tablespoon
Onions, chopped	2 tablespoons
Salt	1/2 teaspoon

PREPARATION TIME: 10 MINUTES

1. Mash chickpeas in a small bowl until they are smooth.
2. Add oil and lemon juice; stir to combine.
3. Add chopped onions and salt.
4. Serve on bread or crackers.

Note: Garbanzo bean is another name for chickpea.

PER SERVING:	
Calories	90
Total fat	4 grams
Saturated fat	Trace
Cholesterol	0
Sodium	148 milligrams

SALADS

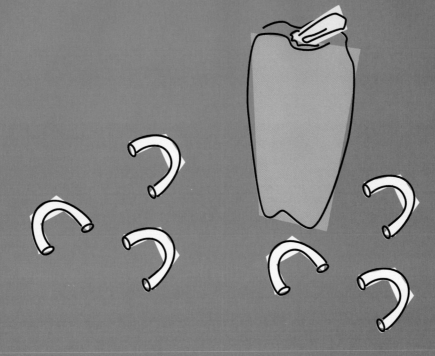

MACARONI SALAD

4 Servings, 1-1/2 cups each

Elbow macaroni, uncooked	12 ounces
Green pepper, chopped	1/2 cup
Salad dressing, mayonnaise-type	1/4 cup
Pepper	1/2 teaspoon
Garlic powder	1/4 teaspoon

PREPARATION TIME: 15 MINUTES
COOKING TIME: 8 TO 10 MINUTES

1. Cook macaroni according to package directions. Drain and cool.
2. Combine green pepper, salad dressing, and spices.
3. Add macaroni and toss lightly. Chill.

PER SERVING:

Calories	430
Total fat	13 grams
Saturated fat	2 grams
Cholesterol	0
Sodium	72 milligrams

ORANGE GELATIN SALAD

4 Servings, 3/4 cup each

Gelatin, unflavored	3 1/4-ounce packages
Cold water	2-1/4 cups
Orange juice, concentrate	3/4 cup

PREPARATION TIME: 5 MINUTES
COOKING TIME: 3 TO 4 MINUTES

1. Place water in a saucepan; sprinkle gelatin over water. Let stand 2 minutes.
2. Heat gelatin mixture until it dissolves (mixture will be clear), about 3 to 4 minutes.
3. Remove from heat; add orange juice concentrate and mix.
4. Pour into 9- by 9-inch pan and refrigerate until firm, about 2 to 3 hours.
5. Cut into 1-inch squares.

PER SERVING:	
Calories	100
Total fat	Trace
Saturated fat	Trace
Cholesterol	0
Sodium	16 milligrams

POTATO SALAD

4 Servings, 1-1/2 cups each

Potatoes, washed, peeled	1 pound (4 medium)
Onion, diced	1 cup
Sweet pickle relish	1/4 cup
Celery, chopped	1/2 cup
Salad dressing, mayonnaise-type	1/2 cup

PREPARATION TIME: 25 MINUTES
COOKING TIME: 15 MINUTES

1. Wash potatoes; place in sauce pan. Cover with water and bring to boil. Simmer until soft, about 15 minutes. Drain and cool.

2. Dice onion and chop celery; combine with pickle relish.

3. Add salad dressing to pickle mixture.

4. Cube potatoes and blend with dressing.

5. Cover and chill several hours.

PER SERVING:

Calories	350
Total fat	24 grams
Saturated fat	3 grams
Cholesterol	0
Sodium	290 milligrams

BREADS AND HOT CEREALS

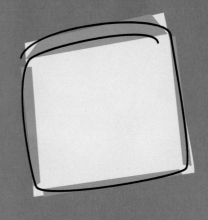

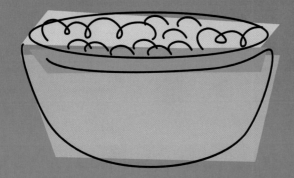

BAKED FRENCH TOAST

4 Servings, about 2 slices each

White bread	8 1/2-inch-thick slices
Eggs	5
Whole milk	1-1/2 cups
Sugar	1/4 cup
Vanilla	1/2 teaspoon

PREPARATION TIME: 15 MINUTES
COOKING TIME: 30 TO 40 MINUTES

1. Lightly grease a 13- by 9- by 2-inch baking pan. Cut each slice of bread into 2 even strips. Arrange bread strips in pan.

2. In large bowl, mix eggs, milk, sugar, and vanilla with an electric mixer on low speed until well-blended, about 5 minutes.

3. Pour egg mixture over bread strips; cover. Chill 4 to 24 hours.

4. Preheat oven to 425° F. Bake until eggs are set and toast is lightly browned, about 30 to 40 minutes.

5. Serve with Cinnamon Sugar Topping.

PER SERVING:	
Calories	460
Total fat	23 grams
Saturated fat	7 grams
Cholesterol	279 milligrams
Sodium	581 milligrams

COOKED RICE CEREAL

4 Servings, 1 cup each

White rice, uncooked	1-1/2 cups
1% lowfat milk	2 cups
Sugar	1/4 cup
Ground cinnamon	1 teaspoon

PREPARATION TIME: 10 MINUTES
COOKING TIME: 15 MINUTES

1. Cook rice according to instructions on the package.
2. Combine warm cooked rice, milk, sugar, and cinnamon. Stir and serve.

PER SERVING:

Calories	250
Total fat	2 grams
Saturated fat	1 gram
Cholesterol	5 milligrams
Sodium	66 milligrams

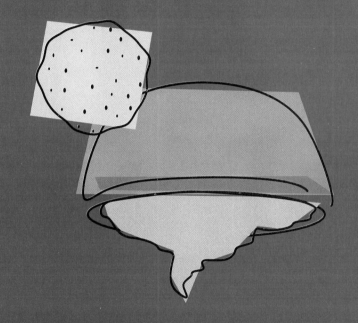

DESSERTS

CHOCOLATE RICE PUDDING

4 Servings, about 2/3 cup each, plus 4 servings for another meal

Whole milk	1 quart
White rice, uncooked	2/3 cup
Sugar	1/2 cup
Semi-sweet chocolate chips	1/4 cup
Eggs	2
Evaporated whole milk	1/2 cup
Sugar	1/2 cup
Flour	1-1/2 tablespoons
Vanilla	1 teaspoon

PREPARATION TIME: 15 MINUTES
COOKING TIME: 30 TO 35 MINUTES

1. Place milk, rice, and sugar in large saucepan. Simmer over medium heat; stir continuously.
2. Reduce heat to low; simmer uncovered until rice is tender, about 25 minutes. Check to make sure rice doesn't scorch. Add chocolate and stir until melted.
3. Beat eggs, evaporated milk, sugar, flour, and vanilla in medium bowl until smooth. Gradually beat egg mixture into rice mixture.
4. Stir continuously; cook over medium heat until thickened, about 5 to 7 minutes. Do not allow pudding to boil.
5. Pour pudding into medium bowl. Cover and chill.

PER SERVING:

Calories	325
Total fat	9 grams
Saturated fat	5 grams
Cholesterol	74 milligrams
Sodium	94 milligrams

OATMEAL COOKIES

4 Servings, 2 cookies each, plus 4 servings for another meal or snack

Sugar	3/4 cup
Margarine	2 tablespoons
Egg	1
Canned applesauce	1/4 cup
1% lowfat milk	2 tablespoons
Flour	1 cup
Baking soda	1/4 teaspoon
Ground cinnamon	1/2 teaspoon
Quick rolled oats	1 cup + 2 tablespoons

PREPARATION TIME: 20 MINUTES
COOKING TIME: 13 TO 15 MINUTES EACH BATCH

1. Preheat oven to 350° F and lightly grease cookie sheets.
2. In a large bowl, use an electric mixer on medium speed to mix sugar and margarine. Mix until well blended, about 3 minutes.
3. Slowly add egg; mix on medium speed 1 minute. Gradually add applesauce and milk; mix on medium speed, 1 minute. Scrape sides of bowl.
4. In another bowl, combine flour, baking soda, and cinnamon. Slowly add to applesauce mixture; mix on low speed until blended, about 2 minutes. Add oats and blend 30 seconds on low speed. Scrape sides of bowl.
5. Drop by teaspoonfuls onto cookie sheet, about 2 inches apart.
6. Bake until lightly browned, about 13 to 15 minutes. Remove from baking sheet while still warm. Cool on wire rack.

PER SERVING:	
Calories	215
Total fat	4 grams
Saturated fat	1 gram
Cholesterol	27 milligrams
Sodium	84 milligrams

PEACH-APPLE CRISP

4 Servings, about 1/2 cup each, plus 4 servings for another meal

Canned sliced peaches, light-syrup pack, drained	20 ounces
Apples, tart, peeled, sliced	2 medium
Vanilla	1/2 teaspoon
Ground cinnamon	1/4 teaspoon
Flour	3/4 cup + 3 tablespoons
Brown sugar, packed	1/4 cup
Margarine, chilled	3 tablespoons

PREPARATION TIME: 20 MINUTES
COOKING TIME: 20 MINUTES

1. Preheat oven to 350° F. Lightly grease 9- by 9- by 2-inch casserole dish.

2. Combine peaches, apples, vanilla, and cinnamon in a bowl. Toss well and spread evenly in greased casserole dish.

3. Combine flour and sugar in small bowl. Cut in margarine with two knives until the mixture resembles coarse meal.

4. Sprinkle flour mixture evenly over fruit.

5. Bake until lightly browned and bubbly, about 20 minutes.

PER SERVING:	
Calories	175
Total fat	5 grams
Saturated fat	1 gram
Cholesterol	0
Sodium	57 milligrams

PEACH CAKE

8 Servings, about 2- by 2-inch piece each

Canned peaches, light-syrup pack, drained and chopped	2 1/4 cups (29-ounce can)
Sugar	1/2 cup
Flour	1 cup
Egg	1
Baking soda	1 teaspoon
Vegetable oil	2 tablespoons
Vanilla	1 teaspoon
Brown sugar, firmly packed	2 tablespoons
Whole milk	2 teaspoons

PREPARATION TIME: 20 MINUTES
COOKING TIME: 30 TO 35 MINUTES

1. Preheat oven to 350° F. Lightly grease 8- by 8-inch pan.

2. Spread peaches in baking pan. Mix remaining ingredients, except brown sugar and milk, together in mixing bowl; spread over top of peaches.

3. Bake until toothpick inserted into cake comes out clean, about 30 to 35 minutes.

4. For topping, combine brown sugar and milk in small bowl. Drizzle mixture on top of cake; return cake to oven, and bake 2 to 3 minutes.

5. Cut into 8 pieces

PER SERVING:

Calories	205
Total fat	4 grams
Saturated fat	1 gram
Cholesterol	27 milligrams
Sodium	171 milligrams

RICE PUDDING

4 Servings, about 1/4 cups each, plus 4 servings for another meal or snack

Whole milk	1 cup
Water	1 cup
Rice, uncooked	1 cup
Eggs	2
Evaporated milk	1 cup
Vanilla	1 teaspoon
Sugar	1/4 cup
Ground cinnamon	1/8 teaspoon

PREPARATION TIME: 15 MINUTES
COOKING TIME: 40 MINUTES

1. In sauce pan, heat milk and water.
2. Add rice, bring to boil, lower heat to simmer; stir mixture every 10 minutes. Cook uncovered until rice is tender, about 30 minutes.
3. In large bowl, mix eggs, 3/4 cup evaporated milk, vanilla, and sugar. Set aside.
4. Add remaining 1/4 cup evaporated milk to rice mixture.
5. Spoon 1 cup of rice mixture into egg mixture and stir. Pour egg-rice mixture into remaining rice.
6. Heat pudding until it boils, stirring continuously. Remove from heat, and sprinkle with cinnamon.

PER SERVING:

Calories	190
Total fat	5 grams
Saturated fat	3 grams
Cholesterol	67 milligrams
Sodium	66 milligrams

SUGAR COOKIES

4 Servings, 3 cookies each, plus 4 servings for another meal or snack

Margarine	1/3 cup
Powdered sugar	2/3 cup
Eggs	2
Vanilla	1/2 teaspoon
Flour	1 cup
Baking powder	1/2 teaspoon
Baking soda	1/8 teaspoon

PREPARATION TIME: 15 MINUTES
COOKING TIME: ABOUT 10 MINUTES EACH BATCH

1. Preheat oven to 375° F.
2. Mix margarine and powdered sugar together thoroughly.
3. Add eggs and vanilla. Beat until blended. Add dry ingredients and blend well.
4. Shape dough into 24 one-inch balls and place on ungreased cookie sheets. Crisscross balls by using fork prongs.
5. Bake until lightly brown, about 10 minutes.

PER SERVING:

Calories	190
Total fat	10 grams
Saturated fat	2 grams
Cholesterol	53 milligrams
Sodium	167 milligrams

FOOD LISTS

The following two food lists show you all of the foods you would need to prepare each week of sample menus on pages 14 to 17 for a family of four.

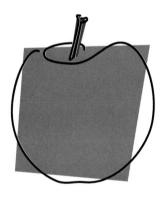

- **IMPORTANT:** The food lists are not shopping lists. Your shopping list will contain only those items that you do not have on hand. Also, sometimes you may need to buy more food than the menu or recipe calls for because of the package size.
- The food lists contain large amounts of nutritious, low-cost foods such as potatoes, macaroni, and rice. Foods with little or no nutritional value—such as soft drinks, coffee, and tea—are not included.
- Depending on where you live and shop and the season of the year, the cost of foods on the lists will vary.

continued

WEEK 1: FOOD FOR A FAMILY OF FOUR

FRUITS AND VEGETABLES

Fresh:

Apples	(6 small)
	1 lb 8 oz
Bananas	(11 medium)
	2 lb 12 oz
Melon	1 lb
Oranges	(26 small)
	5 lb 7 oz
Cabbage	4 oz
Carrots	1 lb 4 oz
Celery	3 oz
Green pepper	3 oz
Lettuce, leaf	4 oz
Onions	2 lb 8 oz
Potatoes	11 lb 14 oz
Zucchini	7 oz

Canned:

Applesauce	2 oz
Peaches	1 lb 10 oz
Pears	13 oz
Green beans	12 oz
Spinach	10 oz
Tomato paste	6 oz
Tomato sauce	1 lb 1 oz
Tomato soup	10.5 oz

Frozen:

Orange juice, concentrate	(8) 12-oz cans
Green beans	5 oz
Peas	5 oz

BREADS, CEREALS, AND OTHER GRAIN PRODUCTS

Bagels, plain, enriched	(8) 1 lb
Bread crumbs	2 oz
Bread, white, enriched	2.2 lb
English muffins	8
Bread, French, enriched	8 oz
Hamburger buns, enriched	8
Crackers, snack, low salt	4 oz
Oatmeal, quick, rolled oats	3 oz
Ready-to-eat cereal (flakes)	6 oz
Barley, pearl	4 oz
Flour, enriched	1 lb 8 oz
Macaroni, enriched	1 lb 11 oz
Noodles, yolk-free, enriched	2 lb 3 oz
Rice, enriched	2 lb 5 oz

MILK AND CHEESE

Evaporated milk	16 fl oz
Milk, 1% lowfat	2-1/2 gal
Milk, whole	3 qt
Cheese, cheddar	8 oz

continued

MEAT AND MEAT ALTERNATES

Beef chuck roast   2.5 lb
Beef, ground, lean 2.4 lb
Chicken, fryer   1.5 lb
Fish
   Breaded portions,
    frozen   1 lb
Cod, frozen   1 lb
Tuna fish, chunk-style,
   water-pack   12 oz
Turkey breast   2 lb 4 oz
Turkey, ground   2 lb
Turkey ham (deli) 11 oz
Beans, kidney,
   canned   1 lb 11 oz
Beans, lima, dry   6 oz
Beans, northern,
   canned   9 oz

Beans, garbanzo
   (chickpeas), canned
            10 oz
Eggs, large   15

FATS AND OILS

Margarine, stick   7 oz
Shortening   2 oz
Salad dressing,
   mayonnaise-type 1 lb
Vegetable oil   9 fl oz

SUGARS AND SWEETS

Sugar, brown   2 oz
Sugar, granulated   1 lb
Chocolate pudding,
   instant   3 oz
Lemonade
   (ready-to-drink) 1 gal

OTHER FOOD ITEMS

(Small amounts are used in preparing the recipes and other foods in the menu, purchase as needed.)

Baking powder
Baking soda
Beef bouillon cubes
Black pepper,
   red pepper
Catsup
Chicken bouillon cubes
Chili powder
Cinnamon
Cornstarch
Cumin

Dry mustard
Gelatin, unflavored
Lemon juice, bottled
Onion powder
Oregano
Paprika
Parsley flakes
Salt
Soy sauce,
   reduced sodium
Sweet pickle relish
Vanilla
Vinegar

continued

WEEK 2: FOOD FOR A FAMILY OF FOUR

FRUITS AND VEGETABLES

Fresh:

Apples   (5 small)
                  1 lb 4 oz
Bananas   (11 medium)
                  2 lb 12 oz
Grapes   1 lb 8 oz
Melon   1 lb
Oranges   (22 small)
                  4 lb 12 oz
Carrots   1 lb
Celery   5 oz
Green pepper   4 oz
Lettuce, leaf   9 oz
Onions   1 lb 4 oz
Potatoes   10 lb 8 oz
Tomatoes   6 oz

Canned:

Oranges, mandarin
                  13 oz
Peaches, light-syrup
                  1 lb 10 oz
Mushrooms   4 oz
Spaghetti sauce   26 oz
Tomato sauce   8 oz

Frozen:

Orange juice,
    concentrate
              (7) 12-oz cans
Broccoli   6 oz
French fries   11 oz
Green beans   1 lb 7 oz
Peas   15 oz

BREADS, CEREALS, AND OTHER GRAIN PRODUCTS

Bagels, plain,
    enriched   (4) 8 oz
Bread crumbs   3 oz
Bread, French,
    enriched   4 oz
Bread, white,
    enriched   2 lb
Bread, whole-wheat 1 lb
Hamburger buns,
    enriched   8
Rolls, dinner, enriched 4
Ready-to-eat cereal:
    Corn flakes   1 oz
    Toasted oats 10 oz
Flour, enriched 1 lb 7 oz

Macaroni, enriched
                  1 lb 5 oz
Noodles, yolk-free,
    enriched   1 lb 2 oz
Popcorn, microwave,
    unpopped   3 oz
Rice, enriched 3 lb 2 oz
Spaghetti, enriched
                  11 oz

MILK AND CHEESE

Evaporated milk   4 oz
Milk, 1% lowfat   9 qt
Milk, whole   4 qt
Cheese, cheddar   2 oz
Cheese, cottage   7 oz
Cheese, mozzarella 1 oz

continued 👉

MEAT AND MEAT ALTERNATES

Beef, ground, lean 3 lb 15 oz
Chicken, fryer 1 lb 13 oz
Chicken, thighs 2 lb 12 oz
Fish (flounder, cod), frozen 2 lb
Tuna fish, chunk-style, water pack 12 oz
Pork, ground 1 lb 7 oz
Turkey, ground 1 lb
Turkey, ham 11 oz
Beans, garbanzo (chickpeas), canned 15 oz
Beans, kidney, canned 15 oz
Beans, vegetarian, canned 1 lb 9 oz
Eggs, large 17

FATS AND OILS

Margarine, stick 15 oz
Shortening 4 oz
Salad dressing, mayonnaise-type 6 fl oz
Vegetable oil 9 fl oz

SUGARS AND SWEETS

Sugar, brown 1 oz
Sugar, powdered 3 oz
Sugar, granulated 9 oz
Jelly 8 oz
Molasses 1 fl oz
Pancake syrup 2 oz
Chocolate chips, semi-sweet 2 oz
Fruit drink 1 gal
Fudgesicles, ice milk 4

OTHER FOOD ITEMS

(Small amounts are used in preparing the recipes and other foods in the menu, purchase as needed.)

Baking powder
Baking soda
Black pepper
Catsup
Chicken broth, reduced sodium
Chili powder
Cinnamon
Chocolate drink mix, powdered
Cumin
Dried onion
Garlic powder
Gelatin, unflavored
Italian herb seasoning
Lemon juice, bottled
Oregano
Paprika
Salt
Soy sauce, reduced sodium
Vanilla

RECIPE LIST

MAIN DISHES

Beef and Pork
Baked meatballs **20**
Beef pot roast **21**
Beef-noodle casserole **22**
Pizza meat loaf **23**
Saucy beef pasta **24**
Southwestern salad **25**
Stir-fried pork and
vegetables with rice **26**

Fish
Baked cod with cheese **28**
Baked spicy fish **29**
Spanish baked fish **30**
Tuna macaroni salad **31**
Tuna pasta salad **32**

Poultry
Baked chicken nuggets **34**
Chicken and vegetables **36**
Oven crispy chicken **37**
Turkey-cabbage
casserole **38**
Turkey chili **39**
Turkey stirfry **40**
Turkey patties **41**

Vegetarian
Cheese-stuffed potatoes **43**

SOUPS
Chicken noodle **45**
Potato **46**

VEGETABLES AND DIPS
Baked beans **48**
Baked crispy potatoes **49**
Potato cakes **50**
Ranch beans **51**
Scalloped potatoes **52**
Shoestring potatoes **53**
Chickpea dip **54**

SALADS
Macaroni **56**
Orange gelatin **57**
Potato **58**

BREADS AND HOT CEREALS
Baked French toast **60**
Cooked rice cereal **61**

DESSERTS
Chocolate rice pudding **63**
Oatmeal cookies **64**
Peach-apple crisp **65**
Peach cake **66**
Rice pudding **67**
Sugar cookies **68**

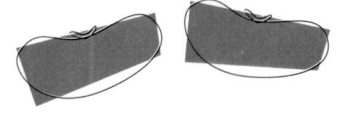

HOW WERE THESE MENUS AND RECIPES DEVELOPED?

The menus and recipes in this booklet show one way to meet nutrition recommendations from the Dietary Guidelines for Americans, the USDA Food Guide Pyramid, and the 1989 Recommended Dietary Allowances. These menus and recipes specifically show ways you can cut back on fat, sugars, and salt on a limited food budget.

The list of foods and amounts used for these menus and recipes reflect the amount of food that could be used for 1 week for a four-person family with two adults and two children ages 6 to 11. Pregnant or nursing women and others with special health conditions may use these menus and recipes also, but may need additional foods or supplements.

ACKNOWLEDGMENTS

We would like to acknowledge the contributions of the staff at the USDA Center for Nutrition Policy and Promotion in the development of this publication. We also wish to recognize the invaluable contributions of the Pennsylvania State University, the contractor that developed and tested the menus, food lists and recipes. Finally, we appreciate the internal reviews conducted by the staff of the Food and Nutrition Service, the USDA Dietary Guidance Working Group, the DHHS Nutrition Policy Board Committee on Dietary Guidance, and the external review conducted by the nutrition specialists with the University of Wyoming, University of Florida, and Colorado State University.

FOR MORE INFORMATION ON NUTRITION

Contact USDA's Center for Nutrition Policy and Promotion. The address is:

U.S. Department of Agriculture
Center for Nutrition Policy and Promotion
1120 20th Street, N.W.
Suite 200, North Lobby
Washington, DC 20036-3406

This publication may be purchased in single copies through the Government Printing Office at (202) 512-1800. Call for price.

Some nutrition materials, including this publication, the Dietary Guidelines for Americans, and the Food Guide Pyramid booklet, may be accessed through the CNPP website at www.usda.gov/cnpp

For additional advice on maintaining a healthful diet, you may contact your county extension home economist (Cooperative Extension System), or a nutrition professional in your local health department, hospital, American Red Cross, dietetic association, or private practice.